KRISTA VALDOVINOS

Postpartum Mommy & Me Mindset

How to Bond With Your Baby, Care for Yourself, and Manage Your Life

This book was professionally typeset on Reedsy.
Find out more at reedsy.com

Contents

1

Introduction

Welcome to the *Postpartum Mommy & Me Mindset*. I'm so excited to share it with you! I hope that you find it useful. This book is for you if you are a new postpartum mother. You may feel a bit overwhelmed and stressed about having a new baby. You may be surprised at the incredible demands being placed on your time. You may not have adequate or sustainable social support. And if you have an especially higher-need baby who fusses a lot, it may feel even more overwhelming. Hang in there, Mamma!

The purpose of this book is to help you navigate the challenging, early postpartum weeks in a way that enables you to care for and bond with your baby, while still taking care of yourself and your other duties. This is not a comprehensive postpartum guide that touches on everything you may face. This is a short, condensed book. It is meant to deliver some useful information without taking up a lot of your time. I know that busy postpartum mothers don't have much time to spare, because I've been there – eight times!

My name is Krista and yes, you read that right. I am a mother of eight.

So I know what you're going through. Motherhood is the hardest job in the world, and I have the deepest regard for all of you mothers out there. Although it's an amazing miracle to welcome a new baby into your life, the postpartum phase is no cakewalk! At times it's exhausting. And sometimes, it's even frustrating.

This book does not focus on the medical aspects of postpartum recovery. Nor will I give clinical advice. Although I have a Biology degree from UC Berkeley, I am not a health care provider. There are other good books available that provide more medically-based information. Instead, I want to share a practical mindset shift that helped me blend the responsibilities of motherhood with other life activities to make a more seamless transition.

One of the toughest parts of the time after birth is to realize your life has completely changed forever, and in a sense, there's a kind of "grieving the loss" of your previous autonomy and lifestyle. You can no longer think solely of yourself, your routine, your own life, your own health, and what you want to do each day. And this is hard. Over the past 25+ years of interacting with other mothers, I've heard a lot of them vent various frustrations that ultimately relate back to the demands being put on their time. They feel like they are not "getting things done," and that they don't have time to take care of their own needs.

So what can a postpartum mother do about this? In this book, I'll be sharing what I did and give some practical ways to apply it. But if I had to sum it up into a small passage that describes my philosophy, it would be this:

Instead of getting frustrated that you're revolving your life around your baby, begin to integrate your baby into your daily activities. Embrace your baby's presence wherever you are and in whatever you're doing. Make as many things as possible Mommy & Me *activities. In short, have a Mommy & Me mindset.*

I'll go into more detail throughout this book. But for now, let's just say that practicing or incorporating the philosophy in the statement above helped me bond with and take care of my baby, while still caring for my own needs. It enabled me to manage my daily duties, with my baby in tow, so I could feel some sense of accomplishment. It allowed me to enjoy my baby and still feel like I was living a life. And during the postpartum phase, this really helped decrease the overwhelm. It also boosted my mood a great deal.

Throughout the book, I will sometimes refer to a baby as your baby, the baby, him, or her. This is just to vary the gender and usage. And before we get started on the *Postpartum Mommy and Me Mindset* ideas, I'll first discuss how some traditional cultures view the postpartum period, how that compares to the more Western culture of industrialized nations, and what I think we can learn from them. Then I'll talk about establishing some reasonable expectations. Finally, I'll explore building a support network. I believe giving postpartum advice isn't as helpful without first acknowledging the importance of a support network. Nobody is meant to do this all alone by themselves.

2

Traditional vs. Modern Cultures

Years ago, I met a woman who was raised in Ethiopia. She met and married an American man and settled with him in the USA.

She told me what the postpartum period looked like in her homeland. She said when a woman gives birth in her Ethiopian community, she doesn't have to do anything for at least a couple of months, perhaps even longer. She explained that other members of the community, like a spouse, family members, and friends, help the new mother. They perform all of her household duties and provide childcare for older children. They also provide all the healthy nourishment and care that the mother needs. In her community, the postpartum woman didn't work outside of the home either. So her only job was to recover from birth, care for herself, and bond with her baby. Wow! That sounded amazing!

There are other traditional cultures that have special care for postpartum mothers. A study in 2007 examined 20 different countries from the following regions: East, Southeast, South Asia, Middle East, Oceania,

Latin America, Africa, North America, and more (1).

This study revealed some common themes in postpartum care in some of the more traditional cultures. Some similarities were they organize support from the community, extend rest periods for the mother, and care for both the infant and mother. This was in contrast to the more Western, industrialized cultures, which were found to focus more on short-term, immediate care and technological interventions. It found that the average postpartum care in Western culture only lasts the first few days after giving birth (2).

Where I live, in the United States, most women do get at least a six-week break from work outside the home. And it can be more (up to 12 weeks unpaid leave) with the Family Medical Leave Act (FMLA). It is also standard to have a postpartum six-week follow-up appointment with a doctor. And some health insurance policies do offer access to nurse telephone hot lines to answer any immediate questions. Our babies also have periodic wellness checks with the pediatricians. So it's not like we have absolutely *no* care at all. However, this type of care is more medical-centered rather than practical in-home care to help the new mother recuperate and transition into her new role. Most women have to be up and about their homes pretty quickly, along with caring for the baby's needs and those of any other children they may have. Fitting in their own needs can be challenging.

Some of us mothers are fortunate enough to have a mother, sister, or an in-law come help us for a period of time. But based on what I've both experienced in my own life and seen with other mothers I know, it's rather short-term – maybe for a few days or a week. The people in our support networks have jobs, live far away, or are just too busy. We're an autonomous society that has grown accustomed to living our own lives. And most of us in the modern, industrialized world no longer live with our extended family or have them nearby. I don't say this to judge it as good or bad. It simply is what it is.

In looking at the more traditional cultures, they do appear to invest a lot of time and care into new mothers to support their healing and educate them on infant care. There's also been a theory that there's a connection between postpartum support (or lack of it) and postpartum mental health. A paper by Stern and Kruckman (1983) proposed that the cultures with very low amounts of postpartum disorders, including "baby blues" and postpartum depression, were the cultures that all had practices in place to provide care and support to new mothers (3). However, this paper was written quite a long time ago. More recent studies propose that there isn't concrete evidence that these traditional practices for postpartum care are connected with the absence of postpartum mood disorders in more traditional cultures (4). Please refer to the cited article in the References section if you want to read more on this topic.

The original hypothesis by Stern and Kruckman seems to be in question and has currently provoked some controversy. Was it accurate at that time in 1983? I don't know. Have outcomes simply changed in recent years? Again, I don't know. But I will say this: Mothers I've spoken with in the modern, Western culture have all expressed feeling some measure of stress and overwhelm during their postpartum period. And they all wished they had more help.

It's common knowledge that too much stress degrades our state of mind. And this can make it challenging to stay calm and think clearly. Therefore, I believe we could stand to learn a few things from the traditional cultures which place a much higher value on postpartum mother and baby care. I suspect that more in-home support for a longer period of time would be beneficial and may alleviate some of the distress for postpartum mothers. That is just my opinion.

Without a cultural protocol for an extended rest period in place, it is also tempting for mothers to feel pressured to get back to "business as usual" rather quickly. At the end of the day, if not much has been accomplished, it doesn't feel so good. And if there's been no time to take care of her own needs, disappointment, or even resentment, can creep in. This is where another practice from the more traditional cultures comes in. And it's one that I *really* like. It's something I learned to incorporate into my daily life so that my baby and I started to bond and blend together more harmoniously.

In traditional cultures, after a mother's prescribed time of rest has passed and she's recovered from childbirth, she resumes her normal daily activities with her baby in tow. In other words, she wears her baby as she goes about her normal work and routine. Whether it's doing domestic work, tending an outdoor garden, or helping with agricultural tasks out in the fields, her baby is strapped to her back, chest, or hip. A variation of this practice is what helped me get through those early postpartum weeks and months. I will explain this in more detail throughout this book.

Now let me be clear. This is not to say that you should never have a break from your baby. In this phase of your life, you are now in a full-time, on-call position around the clock. And you do need breaks. I'm not advocating that you remain side by side for twenty-four hours a day, seven days per week. I'm saying that it may be easier and more harmonious to do things together, as much as your situation allows, so that you can meet both of your needs simultaneously. As you read on, I'll give some concrete examples of what this can look like.

3

Setting Reasonable Expectations

irst of all, prepare yourself with some realistic expectations. A nurse once told me the analogy that giving birth is like running a marathon. After you run a marathon, are you prepared to get right back out there and run another one? No, of course not. How soon do you think you'd want to run another marathon? Probably not very soon. What things would you most need right after running a marathon? Rest, hydration, nourishing food, and perhaps a massage for the sore muscles. That would all be great! Likewise, after giving birth, you do need a period of rest and recuperation.

We are all different. Each of us heals and gains back our energy at our own pace. Some recover more quickly than others. And for those of you who had a Caesarian section, you've just undergone major surgery! So you need even more time to recover. Accept that you will need to slow down for a time, especially during the first few weeks. Please talk to your doctor and follow the advice you are given. Avoid too much physical exertion, and listen to your body as it tells you what it needs.

Accept a disrupted routine, at least temporarily. It won't last forever. I promise! But in these early weeks, just focus on getting your rest and on being with your baby. Babies are social creatures, and your baby will likely want to be close to you much of the time. It's what he or she has been used to for the past nine months while growing inside of your body.

For the time being, let go of the pressure to get things done. Practice some self-compassion and don't be hard on yourself. Remember, it's as if you just ran a marathon. So give yourself a break. Focus on rest and recovery and on getting to know your baby. I will cover the topic of sleep and rest in a later section of the book. For now, let's talk about building a support network.

4

Building a Support Network

Step 1: Brainstorm

Brainstorm ways to enlist some in-home support. This includes getting your partner involved too. But don't stop there, because your partner is also living with the new baby, is possibly still working a job, or may have to return to work soon. With the Family Medical Leave Act (in the USA), both parents can get up to 12 weeks unpaid leave. But many families cannot go without income for that long, requiring one or both parents to return to work sooner.

If your heritage is not rooted in a culture where more long-term postpartum support is customary, then you may need a strategy for getting some assistance. But it's well worth the effort. Because any household support you enlist in the early weeks will improve your chances of getting rest. I'm talking about helpers who will do the real work for you, like chores, meals, rocking the baby if he won't settle down, etc. I don't mean the kind of "pseudo-help" that's really just people who want to come over, hang out to see the baby, and keep talking your ears off. Some relatives and friends may think you're fully ready to entertain them. You don't want that kind of "help." At least not in the early weeks.

In my case, I never had any one individual person who could offer long-term assistance. And you too may be in a situation where you have nobody who can give more than short-term help. So I recommend doing this: compile a list of as many people as you can think of. If you have more than one person answer with a "yes," then arrange for different individuals to come over and help on different dates or times. That way, you will have more coverage collectively. If some of the people on your list don't know how to care for a mother or baby, that's OK. You can ask them for support in other areas, such as household chores, preparing meals, or babysitting any other children you may have. Here are some suggestions:

Volunteer Help

- Partner or spouse
- Mother
- Father
- Sister
- Brother
- Mother-in-law
- Sister-in-law
- Friends from your church community, especially those who don't work
- Close friends in general, who might be willing to take time off work or at least come to offer support on a weekend
- Referrals from your church of retired people who like to do volunteer work
- Retired relatives

- Non-retired relatives who are willing to take some time off work
- Retired neighbors
- Members of any other community or club to which you belong
- Older teen child. When I had my eighth child, my oldest was almost 16. She was able to help with household tasks and some childcare.

Paid Help

- Hired babysitters (young ladies you know or strangers through reputable agencies)
- Postpartum care service companies: doulas, newborn care specialists, nurses

You don't necessarily have to use everyone on your list. And quite frankly, even if you asked all of them, not everyone will say "yes." The hired options are the least likely to decline. But not everyone has the financial means to hire help. If you have no volunteer options and you're on a budget, you can consider paid help for just those days when you feel the greatest need. Many mothers have told me that the first night home from the hospital was the hardest. Others say the first few days at home were super tough. I actually found the first week pretty rough with some of my babies.

Hiring a babysitter could be as simple as paying someone you know in your neighborhood or asking your friend's college-aged daughter. There are also agencies that provide in-home babysitting for your childcare needs, but they do tend to be more expensive than hiring individuals that you know. These local agencies are easy to find through online search engines. Just be sure to look for reviews of the agency and its employees and choose one with a good reputation.

There are also local postpartum care services you can hire. I'll distinguish between two different types. There are postpartum caregivers who are independent contractors and work for themselves. Many doulas fit into this category. A postpartum doula is certified to provide postpartum support to a mother and baby, but will also support other needs within the family. A newborn care specialist focuses more on the baby. There are also organized agencies that employ doulas, newborn care specialists, and in some cases, night nurses or even registered nurses. You will need to do a local online search to see what is available in your area. Check reviews, and if possible, get a referral from somebody who's used the services before.

After one of my births, I used a postpartum doula for a few days. It was a good experience and she offered me a lot of moral support (along with preparing yummy lunches). One added bonus was that she brought her teenage son, who was on summer break, and he spent time with my two young boys to keep them occupied. He also fed them lunch. I personally like the holistic approach of the doulas. They care for the mother, baby, and the family. They are usually trained in breastfeeding as well.

Extra tip: If you find a doula or newborn care specialist who is still in a certification program and trying to gain clinical experience hours, you may be able to hire the doula for very low cost or even for free. Just be sure the doula or specialist has the minimum necessary training completed so they arrive with the basic skills you want.

Step 2: Prioritize Your List

Now that you've brainstormed some ideas, put them in order of preference. You may prefer to start with the volunteer options first, and then move on to the paid options if needed. Then start reaching out to them, one by one. If anyone responds with a "yes," discuss with them which days and times they have available. This is a great job for your partner. You'd probably rather be resting than spending your time talking on the phone or sending out emails to people. I remember my husband reaching out to his retired relatives for me, and his aunt came to our home several times to help me. Eventually, after I had physically recovered, she invited me periodically to her house for lunch. I would relax while she helped with my baby, provided food, and offered moral support. This also became a wonderful way for me to foster a connection with another adult, get out of the house, and lift my mood.

Step 3: Schedule Your Help

Once you know who's willing and available to help you, take out a planner or calendar and schedule the dates and times. As mentioned above, the idea is to get several different helpers that you schedule at different times, so that collectively you have as much coverage as possible. Schedule your greatest times of need first, and then go from there.

5

Sleep

Hands down, the number one concern I hear from new mothers is their lack of sleep. I hear the complaints, "I feel like a zombie," "I'm in survival mode," and "I'm getting NO sleep." Herein lies a dilemma; having just given birth, you especially need rest. But you now have the tremendous responsibility of a baby who is entirely dependent upon you for all of its needs. So what can you do?

Step 1: Check With Your Support Network

If you've been able to establish a support network (as discussed previously), lean on them as much as possible, asking them to cover for you while you rest. Sometimes even small things will help. For example, when I gave birth to my first child, my mother was still working full-time as a school teacher. So she didn't have a ton of time on her hands. But since I lived in the neighboring town, she came over when she could. Sometimes she stopped by on her way home from work for a while. She did things like prepare a meal (to save me time) and rock my

15

baby to help settle her down to sleep. This enabled me to take a nap without any concerns. Whenever you have that kind of help available, take advantage of it.

What if you don't have immediate support available and you need some sleep? Move on to the next step.

Step 2: Try These Mommy & Me Suggestions

- First of all, <u>sleep whenever your baby sleeps</u>, day or night. Make that your new mantra. During the early weeks, most babies don't have a set sleep routine. They simply sleep when they need to, around the clock. Adapt yourself to your baby's sleep habits in the early weeks.
- Whenever possible, sleep with your baby cuddled close to you. Your baby is used to being inside of you, feeling your warmth and your heartbeat. Many babies will sleep better and longer if you simulate the environment they've been used to already. If you are concerned about sleeping close to your baby, check with your nurse or pediatrician about the current recommendations for safe co-sleeping to guard against suffocation.
- If your partner doesn't want the baby in the same bed at night with you two, you can place a bassinet next to your bed as an alternative. There are also special bassinets that attach to one side of your bed. Alternatively, you and baby can go to another room in the house for part of the night. That's what I used to do.
- If you're breastfeeding, learn to breastfeed while lying down. It may take some practice. Latch your baby and let him nurse indefinitely. This is one of the best ways to rest; your baby will feel comfort, and warmth, and even pacify himself at your breast, whether or not he's

drinking much.

- If your baby has trouble settling, use movement to lull him to sleep more quickly. Try rocking, swaying, or walking the floor with your baby. Then lay down with the baby cuddled close to you to hopefully keep him asleep.
- Use white noise, sound waves, music, or singing to lull the baby asleep while he lies beside you. This may simulate background noise the baby heard in the womb. You can search for sleep music, sound waves for sleep, or white noise on a mobile device or computer and listen while sleeping. Sound waves and sleep music may help you sleep better so you feel more refreshed.
- If all else fails, ask your partner to take a shift with the baby after work. Then lie down and take a nap.

6

Feedings

Another common area women have problems with is feeding their babies. Breastfeeding can be challenging, especially for a first-time mom without experience. There are a lot of books on the market about breastfeeding, but I prefer a more hands-on and personal approach. So I used lactation consultants and attended some La Leche League meetings. Since I'm not a certified lactation consultant, I won't be giving the specific mechanics of breastfeeding. You can do an online search for local lactation consultants and La Leche League meetings in your area. Or if you prefer books, you can search for some breastfeeding books on Amazon.

Unfortunately, I struggled with breastfeeding. As it turned out, I had a thyroid condition that affected my milk supply. So when I breastfed, I had to supplement. If you do choose to breastfeed but are struggling with it, don't blame yourself or think you're a failure. I've heard that a lot. I mean a LOT. Many women feel like they've failed if they don't produce enough milk and their baby loses weight. Or they feel guilty about supplementing with formula or bottle feeding altogether.

My advice to you is to get help from the professionals to see if the issues can be resolved. But if the issues aren't fully resolved, don't feel bad for supplementing with formula or for deciding to bottle feed. Have some self-compassion. The last thing you need is to beat yourself up and work yourself into a funk about it. You've got enough on your plate already! You're a great mother however you choose to feed your baby. The important thing is that you are feeding your baby.

One of the hardest things about feeding your baby is the demand on your time. It's one of the most time-consuming tasks of the whole postpartum experience. Whether you breastfeed, bottle feed, or a combination of both, you do a lot of sitting with your baby. And this frustrates a lot of women who don't like sitting still for so long. They feel like they should be up doing things.

Breastfeeding can tend to take longer, at least in the beginning. However, there is the advantage of not having to prepare and heat the bottles of formula, and not needing to wash/sterilize bottles and nipples. That advantage actually saves you time. The exception to this is if you are supplementing and/or using a breast pump. Then there are things to wash. Plus the pumping itself adds to the time associated with feeding.

With all the time you spend on things related to feeding, no matter which method you choose, you may feel hard-pressed to find time to feed and hydrate yourself! So what can you do?

Step 1: Have a Support Person Help With Your Meals

When your partner is home or whenever a support person is over, you can have them bring you your meals. But plan ahead for when there's nobody around to help you. Have your partner or other support person leave you prepared, healthy meals and snacks in the refrigerator that you can grab and go. You can also enlist their help to set up your feeding station (see below). If you don't have someone helping with this, then pre-plan the grab-and-go foods for yourself each day. Move on to step 2.

Step 2: Eat When Your Baby Eats

When your baby feeds, you can also feed yourself. This will ensure that you meet your need for nourishment.

- Plan out where you want to sit for most of your feeding sessions.
- Set up a "feeding station table" ahead of time, next to your seat. Use an end table, coffee table, or extra chair as a storage surface.
- Stock the table with nonperishable snacks and water bottles for yourself. This is also a job your support person can do for you ahead of time.
- If you want a perishable meal or snack from the refrigerator, remember to grab it before sitting down to feed your baby.
- Use the lulls in feeding to nourish and hydrate yourself. Sometimes the baby slows down or spits out the breast/bottle, or falls asleep temporarily. Sometimes he needs a burp or just wants to chill for a minute. During these breaks, you are more likely to free up one of your hands. Use those opportunities to grab some food or water from your feeding station table to nourish and hydrate yourself.
- Of course, you don't have to eat every single time the baby eats. But have everything set up ahead of time in case you do get hungry. And do drink some water often, especially if you're breastfeeding.

7

Hygiene & General Self-Care

When you're so busy with your new baby, it can be hard to do some of your most basic hygiene practices. Things like taking a shower, having skincare and dental care routines, styling your hair, or applying cosmetics seem more like luxuries. But at the very least, you'll want to be clean. Some mothers shower only when the baby is napping. But since it's important to sleep when your baby sleeps, I recommend a different option. You could wait until your partner gets home from work, but I also suggest you try bringing your baby along. Perform your essential cleanliness habits with your baby nearby.

Step 1: Set the Stage

- Take care of any pressing needs your baby may have first. Make sure she's been fed, burped, has a clean diaper, etc. This improves the chances of her being content.

Step 2: Try These Mommy & Me Suggestions

- First make sure that your baby is safely secured from any outside risks, such as pets, other children, or household items (like any items that could fall on the baby) before you step into a shower.
- Secure your baby in a reclined baby carrier or car seat. As the baby gets a little older, you could also use a reclined bouncy seat with a toy bar. Some newborns can also do okay in a bouncy seat for a short amount of time. But check with your pediatrician for recommendations on that. If there's a musical function on the toy bar, that's even better.
- Another option for young infants who don't crawl yet is an infant play mat with hanging toys. Some of these come with musical options too. My babies loved to lay there and stare up at all the colorful hanging items. These play mats are readily available at many stores and online. They are called by a variety of names, such as baby play mat, baby play gym, gym activity mat, baby game mat, etc., and most of them are rather inexpensive. You can place the play mat on top of a bath mat or folded-up towel to provide extra padding for the baby to lay on.
- If your baby responds to music or white noise, play some in the background on your mobile phone.
- Take a shower, or use the sink and mirror to perform any hygiene or self-care that you need. If your baby fusses or cries while you're in the shower, you can peek out, look over and talk to her and reassure her. Sometimes your baby just wants to know that you're there. Playing some music in the room may also soothe her.

8

Household Chores & Routine

For your first couple weeks at home with your baby, ideally, your partner and support people will help with covering a lot of the chores. I've already covered that in the section about your support network. Once you start healing and gaining your strength back, you'll start to resume some of your household duties. You may be chomping at the bit to get things back to "business as usual" and feel lost without a consistent routine. I recommend that you begin slowly and ease into it. Do only what's necessary at first to test the waters and see how you feel. Take your time. There's no hurry or need to pressure yourself. Even completing the smallest of tasks can give you a sense of accomplishment. At least it did for me. I recommend making it another Mommy & Me activity as you resume your chores. I liked to look at and interact with my baby as I kept him near me while I performed household tasks.

Step 1: Set the Stage

- Take care of any pressing needs your baby may have first. Make sure she's fed, burped, has a clean diaper, etc. This improves the chances of her being content.

Step 2: Try These Mommy & Me Suggestions

- Keep chores to a minimum at first, sticking only to what is most necessary.
- Do necessary chores when your baby is awake, so you can sleep when the baby sleeps.
- Wear your baby on your body in a baby wrap or carrier as you do your chores whenever possible.
- Alternatively, you can secure your baby into a reclined baby carrier or car seat and keep him near you as you perform your household duties. This is a great option if your back is sore or if you don't feel like carrying your baby for too long. It's also nice if you'd rather face your baby so you can interact with him as you do your chores.

9

Physical Exercise

This is my favorite Mommy & Me activity. It's so much fun to exercise with your baby! Before beginning an exercise routine, it's best to check with your doctor before physically exerting yourself too much. You want to make sure you're body has recovered and that you don't have any postpartum complications. Prior to my six-week postpartum follow-up appointment, I mainly just took gentle walks, nothing too strenuous.

Many postpartum women suffer from a poor body image. They feel flabby or frumpy and wonder if their body will ever return to their per-pregnancy shape. Some women felt they were out of shape to begin with, and now, after pregnancy, there is even more weight to lose. I would like to challenge you to let go of any one stereotypical body ideal. Try not to place the focus so much on weight, size, or even how you look. Instead, place the focus on your health.

Exercise is so healthy. It improves circulation and increases blood flow throughout your body. It helps your joints stay lubricated. Some forms of exercise build muscle strength, while aerobic exercise can strengthen your heart. If you incorporate stretches, this increases your flexibility. Exercise is beneficial for your overall well-being and makes you feel really good, as long as you don't overdo it. According to the Mayo Clinic, exercise can even increase the release of your body's feel-good hormones, called endorphins, thus reducing stress and improving your mood (5). This last benefit was so helpful during my postpartum phases. I found that exercise really did boost my mood!

Exercise is basically just movement. It can be any kind of movement that you enjoy. I encourage you to choose something that you enjoy, but also something that you can do near your baby, and eventually with your baby. In the earliest weeks, your baby is limited in what he can do, so you'll mostly have him beside you. But as he gets older, you can actually do movements with your baby. As a new mother, I found it so much easier to sustain a regular exercise routine that way. Below are a few starting points for making your exercise routine a Mommy & Me activity.

Step 1: Set the Stage

- Take care of any pressing needs your baby may have first. Make sure he's been fed, burped, and has a clean diaper, etc. This increases the chances of your baby being content.

Step 2: Try These Mommy & Me Suggestions in the Early Weeks

- Place your baby in a wrap or carrier. Go for a walk around your neighborhood are at a local park. You can also use a stroller in its reclined position.
- Place the baby on a blanket next to you while you do some free postnatal yoga videos on YouTube. Your baby can watch you while he's lying on his back. Interact with him periodically.
- There are also postnatal Pilates and other postnatal mat work videos for free on YouTube. Or you can buy exercise programs in a variety of formats: video streaming, DVDs, and books.
- If you want to do more aerobic-style movements (stepping, sliding, jumping, dancing), place your baby in an infant swing or portable bassinet to get him off the floor. You don't want to risk stepping on or tripping over him. Place the swing so that your baby is facing you, and not too far away, so that you can smile at and interact with him periodically.
- The swing also works great if your baby is getting fussy.
- Combine your baby's "tummy time" with getting in some movement for yourself. Your pediatrician will likely recommend giving your baby frequent tummy times. It's great for strengthening a baby's neck, shoulders, and arms (6). It also helps your baby develop motor and visual skills (7). Tummy time needs to be supervised. So avoid using any exercise videos or books during these sessions. Place your baby on his tummy and on top of a blanket or play mat. Sit or lie in front of him. You can vary your position around your baby so he attempts to move his head and body in different directions. While you encourage and interact with him, do some exercises that you've learned by memory. You can do yoga, Pilates, ab work, leg lifts, pelvic tilts, Kegel exercises, or even breathing exercises. Do anything you like. The key is to just get your body moving in various ways.

Step 3: Try These Mommy & Me Suggestions in Later Weeks or Months

These ideas are for babies who are a bit older. You may still continue with any of the activity ideas from the above list. But consider adding some of the following ones too. Please check with your pediatrician if you have any questions about what's an appropriate activity to do with your baby at specific ages.

- Mommy & Me Yoga: Take a class, buy a program, or find free videos on YouTube (about 3-4 months old).
- Mommy & Me Pilates: Take a class, buy a program, or find free videos on YouTube. There's also a book I recommend called *PeeWee Pilates* (about 3-4 months old).
- Take a Mommy and Me swimming class. Although it may not seem like that would be much exercise for you, you really are working muscles as you move through the water against its resistance. This could also be aerobic exercise if you're moving around enough. You'll also be lifting your baby in and out of the water, which works your upper body. If you have your own pool, you can do this at home (about 6 months old).
- If you are a runner, there are specially designed jogging strollers for this purpose. Secure your baby in the stroller and go for a run (about 6 months old).
- Place your baby in a backpack and go for or hike. But be careful about the terrain. You don't want a super rugged or difficult terrain due to the risk of falling (about 6 months).
- Don't forget your baby's tummy time sessions. You can sit or lie down with her during her tummy time and do some body movements yourself. Babies may continue with tummy time throughout their first year (8).

10

If Other Children Are in the Home

I f you have other children in the home besides your baby, it can be a bit more challenging. You need to consider their needs too. The flip side to this is that older siblings are often great at entertaining their baby siblings. And some are skilled at making the baby smile and stay content. Just be sure to supervise the interactions to see how safely the older children behave with your baby. Here are some workarounds for when you have other children in the home.

Step 1: Check With Your Support Network

- Lean on your social support structure, if you have one established, and schedule some outside volunteer help.
- If you have at least one child that is old enough to babysit, (like middle school or older), schedule times when the older sibling(s) can watch the younger one(s). My older children used to take turns watching my toddler, preschooler, and kindergarten-aged children in the afternoon for me.

- Next, consider the in-home paid options, such as babysitters and doulas.

- Finally, explore the options for paid outside options, and ask your partner to provide the transportation (at least for a while). Can you put your child in a daycare facility part-time? Is he old enough for a local preschool?

- If you don't have the means for these paid options, consider some free outside options in your community. For example, there are babysitting co-ops in many communities. You could negotiate with them to reciprocate the babysitting later when your baby is older. I'm not recommending that you babysit other people's children right now.

- Another free option is the public school system preschool. It may also be called Prekindergarten or PreK. Many school districts offer free PreK to children who qualify. Some districts have programs for both 3-year and 4-year olds, and also for special needs education. Check with your school district for the requirements in your area. Criteria can vary, but some examples of eligibility requirement categories to qualify in my local school district are the following: special educational needs, household income, children of a parent who is an active duty member of the military, language issues, and more.

Step 2: Try These Mommy & Me Suggestions

- While you do your chores, give your other children a job. They can help carry the clothes to the laundry room and help place them into the washing machine. They can place clothes into the dryer, or gather toys and baby items throughout the house. You can give them a small broom, duster, or push toy to do some pretend cleaning alongside you. They can bring you the baby's diapers. They can bring you a bottle of water or a snack while you're feeding the baby. The possibilities are endless. In all of your activities, think of ways to include your other children who are at home with you.

- When you sit down to feed your baby, have a play area and maybe a snack area nearby for your other children. Your partner can help you set this up in advance.

- As mentioned before, other children can entertain the baby for a while. But if they are not old enough to be responsible, make sure to supervise.

- Getting naps during the day is perhaps the most challenging issue of all. If you have neither a support person nor outside facility options, then schedule a time when all of your young children lie down to rest. You can have a designated time in the morning and another time in the afternoon, during which you require your other children to stay in their rooms, whether they sleep or not. If any of them still use a crib, it's easier to keep them safe. But if not, make sure the rooms are thoroughly child-proofed and have doorknob attachments that prevent them from exiting the room. Then lie down with your baby, using any tips presented in the sleep section.

- For some children, visual cues may help. Create a visual schedule or chart using simple pictures of important activities. These might include eating, playing, cleaning, or napping. Then coordinate these with your own tasks to make some connections between the flow of your day and your children's activities. For example, if you need to feed your baby, you can tell your other child (or children), "I'm feeding the baby now. That means it's your playtime. Let's go put the toy picture onto your chart, and go to your play area." Or with nap time, you may say, "I'm lying down with the baby now. That means it's your nap time or quiet time. Go put the nap time picture onto your chart, and then I'll take you to your bedroom." As your children begin to see some predictable connections and know what to expect, they're more likely to cooperate with you. If you don't feel artistic enough to create your own pictures, you can cut out pictures from magazines or buy some toddler activity cards. There are also ideas for visual schedules online.

- To increase the chances of cooperation even more, create a reward system for the older siblings. You could use a sticker chart system. Or you could allow them to earn privileges, such as an extra bedtime story, a special outing with dad, or anything that seems appropriate to you. The point is to reward your other children for being cooperative.

- If your other children are very young, save taking a shower for times when they are watched by someone else (a partner, a babysitter, or a responsible sibling) or are secured in their bedrooms. Performing your other hygiene tasks at the sink might be okay with the baby and other children near you, as long as the other children behave safely.

11

If You're Returning to Work

Most of the tips in this book pertain to situations where you're at home with your baby and not working at a job. If you are returning to a job outside of the home, you're probably not bringing your baby to work with you. The exception is if you work for a company that provides on-site daycare. In that case, your baby can be on-site, and you can stop in on your breaks and lunch hour to spend time with her.

For those of you who have your own business or work in a remote position from home, you may be able to keep your baby near you while you work. Having your baby near you while trying to focus on work may not be the best thing for your productivity. But many mothers do it because they don't have other options. And during the pandemic, almost everybody did it. I heard stories of both mothers and fathers working at their computers with a baby on their lap. Apparently, it can be done, although it may not be easy.

Step 1: Check With Your Support Network

Can you get some help at least part of the time, either paid or volunteer? It's especially helpful to have someone else take your child for a little while if you have to be on a call or meeting.

Step 2: Try These Mommy & Me Suggestions

- Keep your baby near you when possible. You can use a portable bassinet, play yard, baby play mat, wrap, etc. You will stay more in tune with his needs throughout your work day.
- If you have to be on a call and need it to be quiet, secure your baby safely in another room until your call is finished.
- If you and your partner work remotely (or are home at least part of the time) you can become a tag team. See if you can coordinate your job duties to take turns managing the baby. That's how my daughter and son-in-law do it.
- If you have older children at home who are responsible, they can take turns entertaining the baby.
- If you have other young children at home in addition to your baby, see the chapter titled "If Other Children Are in the Home" for additional tips.

12

References

1. Dennis, C.-L., Fung, K., Grigoriadis, S., Robinson, G. E., Romans, S., & Ross, L. (2007). Traditional Postpartum Practices and Rituals: A Qualitative Systematic Review. *Women's Health, 3(4), 487-502*
Retrieved on August 25, 2023, from
Traditional Postpartum Practices and Rituals: A Qualitative Systematic Review - Cindy-Lee Dennis, Kenneth Fung, Sophie Grigoriadis, Gail Erlick Robinson, Sarah Romans, Lori Ross, 2007

2. Ibid.

3. Stern, Gwen & Kruckman, Laurence (1983) "Multi-disciplinary perspectives on post-partum depression: An anthropological critique," *Social Science & Medicine*, Elsevier, vol. 17(15), pages 1027-1041, January.
Retrieved on August 27, 2023, from Multi-disciplinary perspectives on post-partum depression: An anthropological critique

4. Stone, K. (2012, October 22). *Is Postpartum Depression Non-Existent in*

other cultures? The FaCTs | POSTPARTUM PROGRESS. POSTPARTUM PROGRESS.

Retrieved on August 27, 2023, from Is Postpartum Depression Non-Existent in Other Cultures? The Facts

5. *Exercise and stress: Get moving to manage stress*. (2022, August 3). Mayo Clinic.

Retrieved on August 26, 2023, from Exercise and stress: Get moving to manage stress - Mayo Clinic.

6. *Benefits of Tummy Time | Safe to Sleep®*. (n.d.). https://safetosleep.nic hd.nih.gov/.

Retrieved on August 28, 2023, from Benefits of Tummy Time | Safe to Sleep®.

7. *What you need to know about tummy time | Tummy Time Tips*. (2022, May 26). Pathways.org.

Retrieved on August 28, 2023, from What You Need to Know About Tummy Time

8. Ibid.

13

Conclusion

Here's a summary of what I've covered: Have realistic expectations for yourself and your baby during your postpartum period. Establish a support network as best as you can. Develop a Mommy & Me mindset; blend your baby into your everyday life harmoniously, and embrace him in whatever you're doing. Live your life, but include your baby. Make as many things as you can become Mommy & Me activities. That way you'll meet both your baby's needs and your own needs. This can apply to sleeping, eating, personal hygiene, chores, exercise, and involving older children. For some of you, it may also apply to remote working situations. You can manage your life and many of your duties with your baby beside you. As a result, you and your baby will bond more closely, and you'll feel a sense of accomplishment.

Feel free to adapt the ideas in this book according to your individual situation. Or pick and choose only the ideas you like. You may even want to think up your own! You can continue this into the later months too if that works for you.

Thank you for reading my book! I hope you've enjoyed it and found it helpful. If you did, then please leave a positive review on Amazon.com describing what you liked about it! Thank you!

You're welcome to reach out to me via email at kristavaldovinos8@gmail.com to ask any questions or to offer additional feedback. Best of luck on your motherhood journey!